21 Ways To Transform Your Health Without Medications

THE COMPASS
HEALTH
TRANSFORMER II

by

Dr Chio Ugochukwu

Published by Compass International.

44546 Orchard Lane, Lancaster CA 93534

ISBN-13:978-1479371723

Editing by Katie Corbett.

Printed in the United States of America.

Disclaimer

This book contains the opinions and ideas of its author. It is solely for informational and educational purposes and should not be regarded as a substitute for professional medical treatment. This is a book for people who want practical suggestions that will help them live healthier and happier lives. No information contained in this book should be considered as physical, psychological, medical, financial, tax or legal advice. The author assumes no liability or responsibility for damage or injury to you, other persons or property arising from the use of any product, information, idea or instruction contained in the content provided to you through this book.

Dedication

This book is dedicated to my lovely wife, Ekene and to my children, Mmeli, Dili, Chiji, Mezu, Nnedi and all those trying every day to transform their lives.

Table of Contents

Introduction

You can start living a healthy life, Right Now! The road to creating a healthy life can be approached in many different ways. You can take the easy way or the hard way. I prefer ways that are simple and easy to implement.

The most effective ways involve making small but significant changes to various aspects of our daily lives. These will involve how we relate to one another, how we eat, how we try to make our dreams come true and how we take care of ourselves medically, physically, mentally and spiritually.

The Compass Health Transformer II will show you 21 easy ways to transform your health without medications. You can begin to implement these in your lives right now with immediate and tangible results. You can create a healthy life for yourself through simple changes to your everyday activities that can help you modify your lifestyle without trying to re-invent yourself.

Let us be honest, with ourselves, we all want to live, healthy, creative and happy lives. This is why most of us try to lose weight by trying different diets and exercise regimen. Our desire for staying healthy is also the reason we visit   our health care providers when we get sick.

The problem with this approach is that we are always playing catch up. Most of us have no idea, what we actually weigh or how much our ideal weight should be, until we fall sick and find ourselves in the emergency room or at a doctor's office.

This is because most of us postpone visiting our health care providers until we find ourselves under a lot of stress or sick. This was precisely what happened to my friend, John, who after many years of "reactive living" discovered he was diabetic, after his second visit for an ear infection.

He was shocked to find out that his limited physical activity and a diet which predominantly consisted of rice, white bread and beef with little or no fruits and vegetables contributed to his diagnosis of diabetes. John was not simply overweight, he was obese.

After the initial shock wore off, John told me he was finally ready to stop "reactive living" in which he merely reacted to events and begin healthy living in which he learned more about himself, anticipated events, and took preventive actions. He told me he was now prepared to eat more healthy foods, even begin to exercise and find a way to lose weight.

Of course, while I agree with my friend, John, on what he needed to do, I also know that most of us need to do a lot more to make our lives more healthy. Though eating well and exercising regularly are important steps in this direction, they are not enough.

I say this, because I have found out that in order to live the healthy, creative and happy lives we all wish for, we need to have a plan that is easy to understand, and easy to implement, yet detailed enough that it covers all aspects of our lives like our relationships and finances, in addition to our health. This is because the triangle of happiness is formed by our relationships, health and finances.

This is where the Compass Health Transformer system and the 21easy ways to create a healthy life comes in. Knowing and using these simple ways will help you to have an integrative approach to healthy living that will show you ways to make the best use of curative medicine, while encouraging you to adapt a healthy life style.

This will help you to make your activities of daily living, part of your comprehensive approach to optimum health.

Use exercise to reduce stress and improve your health

What I have found out from personal experience and from those who exercise regularly is that participating in daily exercise will make you healthier. Exercise can also diminish the effects of stress on your body.

Think of the number of times you have heard someone you know say that the doctor says, "it's stress related". Normally people will laugh it off, concluding that doctors say that when they don't know the real solutions to your problems. The truth of the matter is that too much stress will play a role in many diseases. We know that chronic stress can lead to increased high blood pressure, increased plaques in blood vessels and increased stress hormones.

To help increase your immune system and decrease your stress level, exercise everyday. This can be as simple as walking everyday or as sophisticated as doing yoga at home. "Movement" is the key word here. Keep it simple, bend, stretch and walk everyday. There's really no need to buy any expensive equipment either, as you can implement more movement into your daily routine and reap the benefits.

If you like aerobic exercise, you should grab a partner and "have a blast " with one of the basic aerobic videos. Or, you can simply go out for a walk and enjoy spending time together. As you may have heard, walking really is the best overall exercise you can do for your health. As long as you have a pair of good walking shoes, you'll be fine.

Walking shoes are great because they make walking more comfortable. However do not use their absence as an excuse for not doing your daily exercise if you are committed to one.

As you go through your daily activities, make it a point to walk a little further. One of my favorite tricks for doing this is to park far away from the entrance each time I go to the grocery store or the mall. This will help you take a few more steps everyday. Try it. You will be surprised how effective this can become for you without changing your lifestyle a great deal.

There are several different exercises that you can do to help eliminate the stress in your life. Walking is among the best, as you can easily lose yourself and your troubles by walking. Even if it is just around the block, walking can do wonders for your health. It can also help to reduce your stress level.

If you have a lot of stress in your life, you may want to consider a gym. Working out and then sitting in the sauna is also a good way to relieve tension. If your gym has a pool, you may find swimming to be very beneficial as well, as it helps you to relax.

If you do not like walking or going to the gym, consider going for swimming exercises, joining a dance class or even playing tennis. If you find yourself doing a lot of standing or sitting as part of your job or daily life, consider bending down to pick something up without using a pick up stick or moving the item towards you with your foot when standing.

The bottom line is that if you find any exercise pattern that fits into your life style and do it regularly, you will see that daily stress in your life will reduce.

Use exercise and physical activity to help you sleep better

As we get older we discover that sleep does not come as readily as in the past. Not sleeping well eventually affects your health. One way most people try to deal with insomnia is to take sleeping pills. However, another option is to increase the amount of physical exercise that you participate in during the day. This is one of the key ways to help you get a good sleep at night. The more active your body is during the day, the more likely you are to relax at night and fall asleep faster.

If you doubt this, watch your children. You will find out they sleep the most, when they have been most busy running around and actively playing all day. They get into bed and fall sound asleep.

With regular exercise you'll notice that your quality of sleep is improved and the transition between the cycles and phases of sleep will become smoother and more regular. By keeping up your physical activity during the day, you may find it easier to deal with the stress and worries of your life.

Research and studies indicate that there is a direct correlation between how much we exercise and how we feel afterwards.

You should try and increase your physical activity during the day. The goal here is to give your body enough stimulation during the day so that you aren't full of energy at night.

Your body requires a certain amount of physical activity in order to keep functioning in a healthy manner. It is also important to note that you should not be exercising three or four hours before you go to bed.

The ideal exercise time is in the late afternoon or early evening. You want to make sure you expend your physical energy long before it is time for your body to rest and ready itself for sleep.

You should attempt to exercise at least three or four times a week for a period of 30 minutes or so. You can include walking or something simple. If you prefer, you can include strenuous activities such as running as well.

Along with running and walking there are several other physical activities that you can add to your daily life to increase your level of physical activity. If you are battling insomnia, you'll find aerobic exercise to be the best.

If you discover that you don't have any time to exercise on a regular basis, you should try to sneak in moments of activity into your schedule. Whenever possible, you should take the stairs instead of the elevator, as little things like that will do wonders for your body.

You should also park your car around the corner and walk that extra block or two to get to your destination. As you may know, there are many small things you can add to increase the activity in your life. Your overall goal here is to have a healthy and well balanced life with plenty of sleep.

Reduce your belly fat to make your health better

As you get older you begin to notice a tiny but perceptible bulge in your waist line.At first you try to ignore it because you know, you haven't changed your eating habits or daily routine. Yet the bulge continues to grow.

Most people look at their belly fat as an embarrassing sin of aging. I would encourage you to look at it differently. Ask yourself why the bulge occurred. Knowing why you have the bulge will help you to be more motivated to reduce it or get and improve your health more.

One of the main reasons for my increased belly fat had increased was that as I have gotten older, my muscle mass has decreased and my ability to use up energy has decreased so that the unused energy has been converted into visceral fat in my internal organs leading to my belly bulge.

The second reason my waist line increased as I got older was that I have added new sources of stress. Now that I am older I worry about my mortgage and my children's education which I didn't have to worry about 10 years ago. New sources of stress mean release of cortisol, the stress hormone. Cortisol leads to the distribution of fat into the abdominal area, making a bad situation worse.

Knowing at least these two reasons, you look at your belly fat more like a health marker than a cosmetic problem and will want to reduce your belly fat. You then decide to do something about the bulge only to discover that the bulge is not that easy to get rid off. If you have tried to get rid of your own bulge, I am sure you would agree with me.

In the past three months I have lost 15 pounds by following a simple plan of eating plenty of vegetables and fruits while reducing my food portion per meal by about a third and walking for at least 30 minutes ,at least three times a week. This has not translated to much success with my belly fat which has not changed much in the past six months.

To deal with these two main contributors to belly fat, I have decided to include muscle strengthening activities like playing tennis, doing pushups and jumping rope to my weekly exercise routine. If you are up to it, you could also add weight lifting. Do what you find comfortable.

These muscle-strengthening exercises will help me increase my muscle mass as well as increase my total energy and reduce the amount of excess energy to be converted to visceral fat. One muscle strengthening exercise is tennis. Try it! You will enjoy it.

Quit smoking to improve your health profile

One way to stay away from the nursing home and rehabilitation centers as you get older is to quit smoking now. I still remember the 47-year- old engineer, I saw lying on his hospital bed, dying of lung cancer. I guess he most have seen the fear in my eyes as he admonished me not to smoke or to quit if I had started. He told me had been a chain smoker all his life. You can improve your health profile within 72 hours by quitting smoking.

I had this experience many years ago when I was still a student. Today almost everybody knows that smoking is bad for your health. The idea of quitting smoking is great, but doing it is usually difficult. One way to begin the process is to remember the health benefits of giving up smoking.

One of the biggest benefits is the saving of money. Consider that a one pack-a- day habit can easily rack up a bill of about $35 a week or me. It may not seem like much, but you could use this money to pay for your healthy food choices or pay your phone bill. This is money you could put into paying for a gym membership. Even if you do not spend your money on any of these choices you can put the extra money into your savings. After all, having a good savings account is one sure way to reduce money worries and its related stress.

While the money is obviously nice to save, other huge health benefits that research tells us are that as little as 20 minutes after you stop smoking you will be able to see a difference in your health.

Stopping smoking can help you reduce your risk of

heart problems, stroke, high blood pressure, lung cancer, and even breathing complications. Remember that after quitting smoking you are able to reverse many of the harmful effects that cigarettes have caused, no matter how long you have been a smoker.

For example, if you quit smoking for a period of 5 years, you are no more at risk of a stroke than someone who has been a non-smoker for their entire life. This is huge considering that those who smoke are considered at least twice as likely to suffer a stroke. Additionally, if you quit for 15 years, you can enjoy the same risk of coronary heart disease as a non-smoker. While it might seem strange to enjoy the risk for coronary heart disease, it is much better than actually having coronary heart disease. Taking these small victories for your health is important since you will be able to significantly improve your quality of life.

Not everyone is concerned about the health benefits. If you find yourself more concerned with the money, then focus on what you can save. Ultimately, the reason you choose to quit smoking is up to you. The way you do it will be based on your personality and smoking habits. You need to look at your lifestyle and determine what truly matters for you. If you are more determined to improve your health, then focus your efforts on the health benefits that stopping smoking for good can really have for you.

The good news is that even if you quit smoking because of your desire to save money, you will still get the benefit of a better health.

Manage your emotions well for health improvement

Another way to be healthy right now is learn to manage your emotions better. Most of us find it hard to manage our emotions on a day-to-day basis. Our emotional well-being is very important for our health because feeling good about ourselves reduces our daily stress level and helps to make our interactions with others more enjoyable.

Believe me, there are factors and activities through out day that can affect our emotional well being. These include time management, stress, relationship conflicts, anxiety and anger. The truth is that we all have problems or things we do not do well. I am sure you have heard the phrase "Don't be so emotional." This is misleading because our emotions play a big role on how we respond to our daily circumstances. We need to learn how to be emotional in the right way, by learning to choose when to fight or be quiet.

Sometimes your doctor will give you the best medical advice but makes you feel like a fool, chances are you will not follow through on that advice. In fact I know of many patients who stopped seeing their physicians precisely for the above reason. The danger of course is that such a decision may prove deadly, especially if it leads to accurate but life threatening diagnosis being ignored simply because you did not like the doctor. Choose to 'fight' by getting a second opinion or simply change doctors.

Don't give up on your health simply because your doctor was not being nice to you. Someone once said that expecting life to be fair to us or complaining about people not being nice to us was like "a vegetarian expecting a lion not to attack him or her because they didn't eat meat." It's not going to happen.

One of the best ways we can protect our emotional well-being and, by extension our health is to expect the unexpected. Each one us must find ways to deal with those times when people return kindness with rudeness, fairness with unfairness. Whenever I encounter such situations, I tell myself "the vegetarian-lion" story; and my cerebral hemisphere goes into overdrive to shut down or redirect my limbic system.

You see, it is the limbic part of our brain that decides what sensory inputs are emotional and how our body will respond to them. If we feel insulted, the limbic system might make us want to react with aggression immediately. However, pausing for a moment might allow us to have a more assertive response that enables us to protect our emotional well-being while taking care of the insult.

The key to emotional well-being and good health is finding healthy ways to deal with our perception of our environment. This would include how we deal with our social and physical environment. This includes how we interact with others and how deal with our deepest fears. If we don't get it right, we build up stress that will ultimately affect our sleep, heart and digestive systems. We all know that stress can cause high blood pressure, stomach ulcers and even sleepless nights.

We can empower ourselves to deal with such circumstances by changing our internal dialogue. As an example instead of saying, "I am not going to stay here and be insulted", you could remind yourself that people lash out or say mean things when they feel frustrated, insecure or uncomfortable. Remind yourself that even vegetarians get eaten by lions and do not take such outbursts personal.

One of the ways to empower yourself is to learn your emotional triggers and have strategies to deal with such situations before they arise or as soon as they arise. Self knowledge, which is one of the seven dimensions of the compass health profile, will definitely enable us to empower ourselves and live more healthy lives.

Here are some of the ways we can deal with emotional tensions when it builds while we are talking to another person:

1, Speak very slowly,

2, Do not speak past each other,

3, Reschedule or postpone the meeting,

4, Change the subject,

5, Follow up later,

6, Take a time out,

7, Try to understand the other person's view point,

8, Take a deep breath

9, Go for a walk,

10, Say a few prayers,

11, Learn to love and care for others,

12, Be positive about yourself.

Remember that learning how to manage your problems does not mean you will not have problems. It means you have figured out a way to adjust to and take care of problems when they arise. Being able to do this on a regular basis will

help you to live healthier, happier lives.

Use conflicts to grow and make your health better

One of the advantages of having an integrated mind set is that it allows you to look at conflicts as an opportunity for change and growth. Conflict resolution is a useful tool for your health. It is a skill you can start to use for your daily life immediately. Every conflict, without exception, produces an unparalleled possibility to help you change. It improves our understanding of what is actually happening in our relationship now.

Conflicts can teach us a lot about ourselves and how to become more competent and effective in our communications with others. This tool can also help us avoid relationship minefields because it helps each person to recognize behavior patterns that lead to conflict. It can help us reduce or even cut down on stress.

For these reasons, conflicts can be good for your health and can allow individuals and even some organizations to periodically relieve built up stress and set up newer, better ways to relate to one another. Conflicts help to reveal deep seated but sometimes unnoticed hidden fault lines in relationships. This could be relationships between father and son, mother and daughter, husband and wife.

Long standing conflicts indicate a growing need to change and an increasing resistance to doing so. They expose contradictory social messages, the absence of obvious vision, or the presence of blind spots. They indicate the moment of discovery that one finds out that something isn't working and the need for a fresh approach to fix or transcend it. The determining element in virtually every conflict resolution may be the mindset of the people involved and their desire to end the conflict. .

In a way this a very sophisticated way of saying that conflicts help us to realize the areas in our lives in which we need to change as well as those situations and circumstances that lead to a build up of stress in our relationships. Remember that the triangle of happiness is founded on our health, relationships and finance.

Conflicts help us to see areas in each person's triangle of happiness with chances for learning and improvement. Once individuals decide they want to take care of their conflicts, the rest is simple. The conflict instantly seems unimportant, a minor difficulty to get over, or a challenge to handle collaboratively.

To some extent, our conflicts are due to our differing needs and wants. The husband might want to spend money and the wife might want to save it. At other times, it is between parents and their children. The child's need is to explore, so the street or the cliff fulfills a need. But the parents' need is to protect the child's safety, so limiting exploration turns into a bone of contention between them. Parent's can make this a teachable moment by acknowledging the child's need to explore while encouraging the child to do it in a safer environment.

We all need to feel understood, nurtured, and helped, but the ways in which these wants are met vary broadly because of our different personalities and spiritual outlooks. Recognizing that conflicts are part of every relationship will help us not to take them too personal and use them as platforms for growth and better health.

Learn to cope with negative feelings throughout the day

How we feel affects how we see ourselves and how we interact with others. If we do not feel good about ourselves, we are less likely to do those things that will make us happy and healthy.

For example, being in a bad mood, can make us decide to skip the fruits and salads that we know are good for our health. Worse still, you may feel so bad that you end up drinking and smoking.

Because our feelings are fragile, a lot of unexpected things can quickly change them. Take the case of my friend, Thompson, who told me how he had a bad day because his son's teacher bawled him out for dropping the student off late. Thompson was angry because he had dropped off his son at 7.50 a.m. and school started at 8.00 a.m. He knew he had done nothing wrong.

I was not really surprised by his reaction because for most of us, being falsely accused or reprimanded can lead to strong negative feelings. My friend was still "reeling" when he told me the story, so I told him to calm down and take a deep breath.

I asked him to call the school and find out why they called him. This is usually my first step in trying to deal with sources of negative feelings. I call this clearing up "weed." By this I mean get as much detail as possible to find out what happened. I told him that as long as we are alive and functional, anything that happened could have been worse. I also reminded him that everything happens for a reason.

If you are dealing with negative feelings, going through these thoughts will help to find much more positive thoughts. Positive thoughts will lead to positive action.

In the case of my friend Thompson, the school officials apologized to him because the wrong student had been identified. He is now all smiles and has promised to always seek the positive in every situation.

Find balance in your daily life

Finding the balance we need to live healthy is not easy for most of us. Although balance is desired, it is hard to achieve because we are discouraged by the pain necessary for change and growth. One of the reasons this happens is that we look at the magnitude of the change desired instead of the small steps we can take to achieve the balance we need for growth in our lives. A journey of a thousand miles, after all, begins with a step.

According to Onyx Ifemembi, the reason most people do not change is because they live stressful lives without balance. It is like sitting on a stool with unequal legs. Granted one can stay balanced for sometime, but if one leg continues to get longer than others, eventually a tipping point is reached and a crash occurs. This means that without balance we cannot live a healthy life.

The "Onyx Stool" is a metaphor for how balance in life is like standing or sitting on a stool with three legs consisting of finances, relationships and health. Most of us get so caught up with work and career (finances) that other legs of the onyx stool do not grow as well. This leads to an imbalance in finances in the Onyx Stool and leads the stool to tip over and fall. Imbalance in our lives can also lead us to tip over and fall. This type of imbalance leads to stress. This stress and imbalance affects other aspects of our lives like our relationships and health.

Stress builds up because our expectations become less than the results that we get. We expect good relationships, but we put 80% of our energy and time into our work. We allow ourselves to be defined by our work. Jesus was a carpenter but

Jesus was defined by his spirituality and relationship with others through which He radiated balance and mastery of life.

Martin Luther King is remembered today not because he was a minister but because he found balance in his life through his spirituality and relationships. He helped us to look beyond skin color and ethnicity in our relationships. If we spend 80% of our time, energy and thoughts growing one leg of our "onyx stool", without cultivating the growth of other legs, we will lack balance and emotional well-being in our lives.

This will lead to a build up of stress and illness in our lives. We shall find ourselves quick to anger and less tolerant of others and their mistakes. We shall find ourselves less able to concentrate and enjoy the simple pleasures of daily life.

How much balance do you have in your life? Is your triangle of happiness balanced? To find out how much balance you have in your life spend fifteen minutes of your day, examining how much time you spend on your finances, relationships, and health . This type of examination is an important aspect of self knowledge which is important for your growth and spiritual health.

As an example if you have eight hours for work, which is part of your finances, and four hours for your relationships you may have an imbalance. This type of imbalance can be made worse if you allow your work to take two hours of your time for family relationships. Your work will grow, but your family relationships will suffer because you have taken 50% of your family time and given it to your work.

Part of the reason this happens is because you have failed to deliver on expectations. Remember when expectations fail to match results, stress arises. The "Onyx Stool" will help us to identify the legs that are over growing as we seek to find balance in our lives, so that we can make modifications that will enable us to grow without crashing.

This is only the first step in our trying to find balance in our lives. It is an important first step because it allows us to examine all three legs (finances, relationships, and health) and determine which aspects require more time and improvement.

Balance in life is also essential for healthy living because once it is absent, stress builds up. The Onyx stool is one of the concepts or metaphors we use in the Compass health transform system for healthy living to help people develop and maintain balance in their triangle of happiness.

Change the negative patterns that dominate your life

It is now an accepted notion that a person's social life can have a big impact on the state of his or her health or happiness. People who spend a lot of time being social have a healthier and longer life than those who keep themselves isolated. This is another of those changes that is always possible to make. Try to find activities that you enjoy and that allow you to socialize.

Make an inventory of the past 72 hours of your life and see the situations and circumstances that predominantly make you unhappy. These are negative patterns that lead to stress, emotional tension, poor emotional control and unhappiness.

A common pattern, I had to overcome was "list overloading" By this, I mean the tendency to list too many things I wanted to do everyday. Sometimes I had a long list like 10 things, without taking into account how long each item would take.

The end result would be that halfway through the day, I would realize that I could not get all I wanted to do, done. This had the effect of making me feel bad about myself. I would begin to feel that I had not worked hard enough to accomplish the simple tasks I set for myself just for one day.

I would get stressed out and feel that the only way out would be to take a time out and eat some food. Yes, eat some food to relax! In such negative moments, I just grab a soda and some snacks which I just gobble down my throat to help me feel better.

Well, you can imagine how that has helped my "healthy" eating plan. It took me a while to realize that the problem was not the soda and snacks, but it had more to do with my emotional stress resulting from my poor planning for the day.

These days, I make my list for the day and attach a time frame to how much time I shall put into each block of activity. I also divide my list into non-urgent, urgent and immediate projects. Immediate projects get done first and others follow.

This approach has helped me cut down on the emotional stress that my past pattern of negativity generated. It is a welcome experience because it has helped cut down on my episodes of emotional eating.

According to a study from the University of Alabama, those who ate in response to an emotional stress-were 13 times more likely to be overweight or obese. We all know the additional health risks associated with being overweight.

The advantage of recognizing the patterns that dominate your life negatively is that you can either change them or be better prepared to respond to such stressors when they occur .While you are in the process of changing these negative patterns that dominate your life, create an automatic response that you can use in such situations without having to eat food.

An example would be to chew bubble gum, when you feel emotionally stressed instead of drinking soda and taking snacks. If you do not like bubble gums, drink water or eat an apple.

Make your daily meal more healthy within 72 hours

The problem we all face when it comes to changing the makeup of our daily meals is that we eat food with a large amount of fat that makes such foods very tasty. This is why most people do not try to make the change. However, if you really want to live a healthier life, you need to find a way to do it. Here are a few ways you can make your meals more healthy within 72 hours.

Start by drinking a glass of water before each meal. This will help you expand your stomach and make you feel full, without eating as much as before. This approach will make you feel full when you are actually 80% full.This is important because eating only up to 80 % full was one of the common practices of people of Okinawa in

Japan,who have the highest number of centenarians in the world.

Another good tip which you can easily implement within 72 hours is to start eating a variety of foods per meal or per day. Eating a colorful variety of fruits and vegetables per meal will help you make your meals more healthy.

Whatever you decide, start small. Remember that little drops of water make the mighty ocean. This thought will help you, even when you feel overwhelmed by the thought of changing your eating habits. When I changed my eating habits, I started by making small changes like adding salads to every meal of rice that I had. I found the whole idea difficult initially but I had to remind myself that I did not want to spend my golden years, chronically ill and being moved from one hospital to another. I took time to find the combination of fruits and vegetables that worked best for me.

Once you begin to add fruits, vegetables and other food varieties make sure you make enough adjustments to make your meals healthy.The characteristics of healthy eating include the following:

Variety-Do not eat the same meal day in day out

Adequacy-Provide sufficient essential nutrients

Moderation-Cut down on too much unwanted constituents like fat, sugar and salt

Balance-Do not let a food type dominate your meals,-too much beef or bread.

Calorie control-Eat enough energy to maintain your preferred weight

Another way to begin to make your meals more healthy is to halve your intake of all pure or added fats. It allows you to reduce your calorie intake because fat has 9 calories per gram, while carbohydrates and proteins have 4 calories per gram. Use half as much butter or spread on your bread, toast, muffins and potatoes; half the usual amount of mayonnaise or sauce on your salad; and half the oil in the pan every time you have to fry. Grilling is better than frying, and always aim to use unsaturated oils like corn, cranola, and olive oils for cooking.

To make your meals healthier eat chicken, fish, beans, cottage cheese, or low fat yogurt. Have eggs, nuts and red meat occasionally but not every day. When you eat chicken or turkey, use only skinless since most of the fat contained in this type of meat is contained within the skin. Reduce the fat content in your milk products. If you are currently drinking whole milk, reduce to 2% fat; from 2% reduce to 1%. Choose lower-fat cheese and yogurt. When you buy yogurt, also check that it does not contain sugar. The good thing about reducing to 1% fat milk is that it remains tasteful.

Plan your meals and snacks ahead of time. Take time to plan at least one lunch and dinner every week without meat or cheese. Build those meals around whole grains, vegetables and beans to increase fiber and reduce fat. If you have something to chew on, get some fish or tofu. You can make every Friday your fish meal day.

Have at least three to five servings of fruit every day. This can be for dessert or snacks. Choose fruit that is in season. One fruit, I like a lot is apple. My rule is to take an apple per meal. If you can, go for those red delicious apples because they contain pectin, a fiber that helps to promote healthy cholesterol levels and contain more amounts of antioxidants than many other types of apples.

Drink water instead of sodas, juices, milky drinks or alcohol. Avoid diet soda - the sweet taste only encourages you to crave sugar. Hot water with a slice of lemon can be very refreshing in the morning. Aim to drink about six to eight glasses of water everyday.

Before you eat any food read its nutritional facts. This will tell you whether the food has a lot of sugar, saturated fat or trans fat, or sodium per serving. Did you know that we only need about 2300 milligrams of salt everyday? This is equivalent to one flat teaspoon of salt. You can learn more about why reading your nutritional facts is good for your health in the next chapter.

Read your nutritional facts for better health

The nutritional facts of any food product is usually found on the label on the outside or side of most food containers. If you are confused about how to use the nutritional facts, I will share a few ideas and examples with you.

In the nutritional facts table, food contents in a package or container is divided into a serving size and calories and nutrients per serving. The nutrient contents are divided into total fat, trans fat, saturated fat and unsaturated fat.

In addition, you can look at cholesterol, sodium and potassium content. You can also learn total carbohydrate content, protein, dietary fiber and sugars.Other food contents included are vitamins and ingredients.

The first thing I do when I read the nutritional facts in a food product, is to look for its serving size.This will help you to quantify the contents in each food you eat.

For example, if a can of Sprite has a serving size of one can and it contains 140 calories per serving then it means you have to drink the whole can to get 140 calories. Compare this to a loaf of bread with a serving size of one slice of bread, and 70 calories per serving size.This means two slices of bread will give you 140 calories.

In this example, by looking at the nutritional facts, you learn that by eating two slices of bread, you get as much calories as from one can of Sprite. As you can see, using the nutritional facts, we can realistically compare contents of two different food products.

Remember that in addition to actual contents in grams and calories, contents are also recorded as percentage daily values based on a 2,000-calorie diet.

Generally, when I look at my nutrition facts, I also look at my sodium, fiber, and fat content. I know people sometimes ignore their sodium content, thinking it does not really matter. Well, it does. Remember the example I just gave you. Comparing a loaf of bread with a can of soda, you find that a single serving of bread contained 150 milligrams of sodium, while the can of soda contained 65 milligrams of sodium per serving size. Can you believe it?

Now if you intend to eat about 1500 milligrams of sodium per day, and start your day with ten slices of bread, you have just eaten 1500 milligrams of sodium to start your day. Then any other sodium you eat for the rest of day will be in excess of your target.

If you enjoy eating bread because of its fibers you may unwittingly be eating too much sodium. Failing to read or use your nutritional facts is like eating without keeping nutritional balance.

Remember that balance (avoiding over emphasis on any type of food or nutrient at the cost of excluding or minimizing another significantly), is one the five components of healthy eating.

The other components are;

*Adequacy

*Calorie control

*Moderation

*Variety

You can more easily achieve nutritional balance and calorie control if you learn how to read and use your nutritional facts while eating.

Eat your food slowly

Even if you did all the modifications to make your daily meals healthy but ended up eating fast, you will end up over eating. Eat slowly. The body is slow to register when you are full and it is easy to eat too much if you are racing through your meals. You can easily do this if you eat and do other things at the same time.

Here are a number of ways people eat and do other activities at the same time that could make them not eat slowly:

*Eating and watching TV. If you eat and watch TV you do not pay as much attention as you should to your food so you end up eating fast and shoveling your food down your throat. Try as much as you can to switch off the TV when you eat. That includes snacks as well as meals. Studies have proved that we eat larger portions in front of the TV, probably because we are much less aware of what we are eating.

*Eating and driving. Most people do this, especially after buying fast food. However it is difficult to eat slowly, when you are concentrating both on eating and following your driving directions. What invariably happens is that we gobble our food our with little or no chewing.

*Eating and talking on the phone will make you eat your food fast. This too, is an avoidable distraction that helps to reduce your concentration on the actual chewing and eating of food.

*Eating and working is another habit that makes you eat your food in a hurry instead of slowly. This is a very common practice among handy men. They pick up their hamburgers and chew their food while they hammer nails into the wall. Two problems here are poor digestion and more accidents or injuries.

Choose food that you can chew. Again this will increase your fiber intake, and the act of chewing will make you feel more satisfied too. This means eating fruit instead of drinking juice. If you have soup, make sure it is chunky.

Another way you can get yourself to eat more slowly and enjoy your food more, is to find a place where you eat on a regular basis everyday. This could be eating breakfast at home, instead of in your car. If due to your busy schedule you cannot do this in the morning then make it your super. Instead of sitting in front of the TV after work ,eating and watching TV, sit at your dinning table and eat your super slowly.

Examine your eating pattern

Make a list of what you eat over a 72-hour period. Get pen and paper write down what you eat for breakfast, lunch and dinner. Be specific, write down whether you eat cereals, rice, potatoes, yams, "garri", pizza, noodles, eggs, chicken, pork, turkey or corn.

Make a detailed list that also includes how much soda you drink, how many cups of water you drink and how much fruits and vegetables you ate. Then you will be able to examine your eating pattern.

The advantage of doing this is that you will quickly find out which type of food dominates your meals. When I examined my eating pattern, I found out that I ate too much beef and rice, with little or no fruits and vegetables. I also found out I ate too much white bread and butter.

When I did this a light bulb lit up in my brain. I finally understood why my last health check had shown that my good cholesterol was low. Good cholesterol (HDL-High density Lipoprotein) protects against heart disease. I had to take action and I did.

I switched to whole wheat bread, which contains much more fiber than white bread and I stopped adding butter to my bread. In addition, instead of eating just white rice, I started eating brown rice. Brown rice has more fiber and more energy.

To increase my intake of fruits and vegetables, I started eating every rice meal with salads consisting of cabbage, carrots, broccoli, spinach and tomatoes to mention a few. Remember, the old saying, "An apple a day keeps the doctor away." I modified it. I started eating an apple a meal. I found out that "An apple per meal keeps you healthy for real." Try this, you will feel great.

As you can see, just by taking the time to examine my pattern of eating, I quickly found things I could do to make my meals healthier without feeling like if I had to completely re-invent myself. Also examining your eating pattern helps you to identify your eating cues or situations that lead to eating more or eating in an unhealthy way.

Studying your eating habits is one of the important pillars of the Compass Health Transformer way to healthy living. Taking small positive steps will help you to modify your eating and living habits without making you feel violated or humiliated.

I am sure you can also examine your own eating habits and make changes. If you try it and have some trouble sorting yourself out, visit us at www.compasswellnessinstitute.com and we will be more than happy to help you.

Question cultural explanations

Every culture has its traditional breakfast. For some, it is bacon and eggs. For others, it is eating high carbohydrate foods like rice or bread in the morning. Do not let cultural norms define your eating habits. You do not have to wait for a Florence Nightingale before you can change your eating habits.

Florence Nightingale was a British nurse who came to Nigeria in the early 20th century and helped to stop killing twins where, it was culturally acceptable in some parts of the country to kill twins. Yes, kill twins! Now is anybody going to tell me that it is right to kill twins. No!!. Just because something happens or is acceptable in a culture does not make it right.

I say this because every culture has foods that seem okay for certain situations and celebrations. In America, turkey is for Thanksgiving. The point I am making is that just because there are traditional ways of cooking and eating turkey for Thanksgiving does not mean, you cannot find healthier ways to eat turkey. One simple way to do this is to eat skinless turkey.

In some African cultures only men were allowed to eat the most choice parts of a chicken. Questions and ease of access to chickens in modern life have led to the death of that tradition. Now men and women can buy and eat chicken as they wish in most African countries.

Remember, your health is your responsibility. Find ways to modify those eating cultural norms without being dismissive. Do you really have to eat candies during Halloween? Do you think if you grew up getting candies every Halloween, you would suddenly stop taking them in your middle age? What about the damage all those years of eating candies would have done to your teeth? Can you teach yourself and your kids healthy alternatives now?

In some cultures and societies the most desirable foods are beef, rich in protein and fat, that has been fried. This is then eaten with pounded yam and soup made from palm oil. In other cultures it is steak or babercues. These types of food will help to build up your cholesterol level and make you more predisposed to heart disease. You have to look for healthy alternatives. Question cultural explanations and conventional wisdom that are not good for your health.

Remember when it was culturally acceptable to smoke cigarettes everywhere. Now you cannot smoke cigarettes in bars, planes, airport terminals and office buildings. If you have forgotten, watch movies from the 1930's to the 1970's. What if you were one of the few to have questioned the cultural norm of smoking everywhere? You would have tried to protect your health even before the policies that banned smoking became the law.

Today, everybody knows about second hand smoke and its related health hazard, so that even in some families, smokers have to go outside to smoke. For the good of your own health, do not go along with food choices that will not be good for your health just because people from your culture may challenge you or make fun of you. Your culture is supposed to help you, not to kill you. You can do this by finding a way to eat right within your culture.

Find a way to eat right within your culture

Find a way to eat right within your culture. This means finding ways to make adjustments to eating habits that you grew up with, without going crazy by trying to count calories. This is a simple but effective approach to eating right in a culturally sensitive way. Different cultures have their dominant food types and specialties which the population of the culture eats regularly.

The dominant or staple food in Asia is rice. In Africa people eat a lot of "fufu" or pounded food like cassava and yams. In Italy it is pasta, in America people eat a lot of pizza and other fast food like hamburgers, fried chicken and French fries.

The simple weight loss plan that is culturally appropriate basically allows one to stick to foods they are used to while adjusting their servings or portions and physical activity instead of their calories directly. This is a more natural approach, in the sense that it encourages one to modify a given eating pattern.

Assuming you need to lose 10 kilograms or 25 pounds, as an example. The first step to take would be to cut down the servings or portions of your regular meal by any ratio you find convenient. For this example let us use about half or a third to reduce your energy intake. This will encourage eating a little less at a time. If you feel pangs of hunger, drink plenty of water or take some fruit. Please do not take soda for water.

The more your servings are reduced, the more weight you would loose. This makes sense since less food intake means less energy intake. The short fall in energy will be obtained from body fat resulting in weight loss. However, reduced servings may mean more hunger pangs. To deal with this, eat more fruits, vegetables and fibers as fillers. Fibers are especially good for your system because they help to increase bowel movement. This has the added effect of making your digestive system more efficient.

In the example above, if reducing your food serving by half for a month has resulted in a 5 pound weight loss, then doing this for a total of five months would result in a total loss of 25 pounds. This allows one to loose weight in a culturally sensitive manner.

For different cultures and settings, different modifications to familiar eating habits can be made. In America this would entail cutting down on fast foods, soda and other processed foods. In a developing country like Nigeria, it would involve cutting down on traditional "fufu' sources like cassava and yam and trying out new things like plantain and wheat "fufu".

Create your own laughter time

Create your own laughter time to deal with stress in your everyday life. You can decide the best time for you to do your laughing. You can consider it your "laughter time out".

A common question I get, when I tell people about "laughter time out" is "how do I laugh during that period?" Think of all the activites that made you laugh in the past and in the past 72 hours. They could be your past mistakes or funny family accidents.

The benefits of laughing are many. It helps you feel good about yourself. It lifts your mood and helps to lower your stress level and blood pressure.

Creating five-minute periods of "laughter time out" loosens tension and uplifts our moods. You can do this at end of the day or during the middle of a heated argument with your spouse, friend or colleague. This will give you a chance to step back and remind yourself that "It could have been worse."

I share this idea with you because I have found it very useful in the past. It has stopped me from going off on a tirade on a number of times and saved my heart and lungs form the consequences of the hormonal surges.

Laughter is indeed the best medicine. Laugh a little, laugh often, it will make you feel good about yourself and reduce the chances that you will engage in negative health activity like binge drinking or eating. Emotional eating can lead to over snacking and can hinder you from keeping off weight even after having a good start.

This was precisely what happened to Tom, a 40-year-old grocery store manager who started gaining weight after he lost his job. He was baffled by his weight gain because he had not changed his diet in the past three years. When he came to see me with his concerns, I found out that one activity that had changed in the past three months of his life was that he had little time for laughter these days.

It turns out that when Tom worked, he used to come home from work and play around with his kids. It was all fun, games and laughter. This usually occurred about 30 minutes everyday.

Sadly after Tom lost his job he found himself spending less time with his kids. Inadvertently, he also cut down on his laughter time. I told him to go back to having a laughter period with his kids. I encouraged him to find out from his kids the fun and funny activities and events that happened to them everyday.

Initially, Tom said he could not to do it every day because his self esteem was down following his job loss. I encouraged him to set aside one day of the week for everyone in the family to share with others the seven funniest things that had happened to them over the week. Reluctantly he did.

Four weeks later, Tom told me he had found his joy back. He said he started feeling better after he and his whole family spent about 1 hour every Sunday, listing their seven funniest activities for the week. He was surprised to find out that having this laughter period helped him to feel good about himself, though he still had no job. This helped him stop over-snacking which helped control his weight gain.

In addition to getting his weight under control, Tom became more confident and he slowly regained his self esteem. He became more positive about the future.

You too can use the funniest events of the week to create your own "laughter time" period and make your life healthier.

Use multivitamins to support your healthy habits

Take your daily multivitamin supplements but do not let them replace your healthy habits. For example take your omega 3 and 6 fatty acids which have been proven to be very helpful for the heart. However do not give up on fish just because you take Omega fatty acids.

According to Wen-Ben Chiou, Ph.D, a professor at Sun Yat-Sen University, "taking dietary supplements increases perceived invulnerability." He reported this in a study in psychological science that found that the assumed benefits of multivitamins may lead some people to cut corners on their healthy eating habits and daily exercise routine. Please, don't do this.

Remember that the foundation of healthy living is forming and maintaining good relationships and habits that will help you deal with daily stress. and unexpected life events. Do not forget "He who fails to prepare, prepares to fail."

Taking your multivitamins should not stop you from going for your regular medical check up as recommended for your age group and family history by your doctor or health care provider.

Find out what you need to do and then do it. If you need to get vaccines, get your vaccines like the flu vaccines. Do not just say you are taking vitamin C and refuse to take vaccines and exercise. If you need to bundle up because it is cold, do it. Wash your hands frequently to minimize your chances of getting an infection.

It is a huge mistake to assume that simply because you use multivitamins you will remain perfectly healthy or suffer only mild illness. Remember that vitamins are usually supplemental and your taking daily multivitamins will be most effective only if you continue to eat healthy, exercise regularly and continue to manage your weight and the sources of daily stress in your life.

Eating right, means that in addition to taking multivitamins, you also make sure you eat fruits and vegetables. The good thing about this, is that through fruits and vegetables, you will also get phytochemicals and fiber in their most natural form.

The conventional recommendation in this regard is to eat at least five servings of vegetables and fruits per day. One way to do this, is to eat plenty of fruits and vegetables servings, per meal every day then use fruits like Persian cucumber or apples for snacks. This can easily get you to the five servings per day goal. Another way, you can increase your fruits and vegetables intake would be by making half of the plate in each meal filled with fruits and vegetables or taking an apple per meal.

Eat your fruits and vegetables every day, but make sure you start your day with your daily dose of your preferred multivitamins without allowing them to supplant the healthy habits you have acquired or are in the process of acquiring.

For example, we know that vitamin B can be found in fish, meat, orange juice and fortified cereals, yet we also know we do not always get to eat enough of the food types I have just listed. If you combine trying to eat right with taking your vitamins, you would end up regularly getting enough vitamin B in your body. This is an example of how you can use vitamins as a health supplement.

Why are B vitamins so important? Because they help to lower the level of homocysteine in blood vessels, which at high levels can lead to damage of the lining of arteries and could lead to a faster formation of blood clots.

Do not let yourself gain back the weight you lost

Measuring your weight regularly is one of the easiest ways to monitor your healthy living goals. Ideally, if you eat the right balance of carbohydrates, protein and fat, you will get enough nutrients and energy into your system without gaining weight.

Of course, we all know that life happens. You start with your own individual health plan as recommended by the Compass Health Transformer, then after a few weeks or maybe even after a few months, you discover that all the weight you lost has been regained. What will you do?

Here are a few tips. First, remember to do your 72-hour life activity review to find out if there is anything bothering you in your relationships, health, or work. If you are diabetic and you do not know it, you cannot effectively address your weight problem until you see a specialist for your diabetes.

If you are very worried about your job or business, you may find yourself doing a lot of emotional eating due to the related stress. This kind of stress is difficult to deal with, but you can always start with a plan to deal with your work and job prospects. One way to do this is to go back to school, get another job or start your own business.

All things being equal, if you discover that you have been gaining weight back simply because you couldn't stick to your individual health plan, then here are a few more tips for you to consider.

A lapse is not a relapse. A mistake is not a failure. If you find yourself not sticking to your fruits and vegetables, think about trying out new fruits you have not tried in the past. Talk to your support group, and share your ideas on eating time and food variety. Try again if you do not succeed the first time.

Finally, do not forget to talk to your doctor or health care provider about your medications. Make sure you are not taking any medications with weight gain as a side effect. This is important yet, it is something that most people forget to do. It is also critical to ask about other medical conditions like thyroid disorders or hormonal imbalance.

Join a healthy living group

Do not try to do everything by yourself. Join a group or form one. This is because no man is an island. It does not have to be a formal group. It could easily be a group made up of family members or friends. Believe me, it is a lot of fun when the whole family is involved in healthy eating and healthy living.

Making everybody in your family a part of your healthy living plan is a great idea. If you tell your children that you are going to eat apples after every meal, and you do not, they will ask you about it and keep you accountable.

Another benefit, you get out of this, is that you start getting into the act of eating healthy. It will be easier to buy milk with reduced fat and get the whole family to eat small carrots and promongrenates.

The next people you need to get into your group will be those in your office whom you share a lunch break with. This way when you think of going for soda, candies and cookies, you will have someone reminding you that you have decided to eat fruits and vegetables during your lunch break. A salad is also a good way to go.

Depending on your budget and personality, you may want to try more formal groups than ones I have mentioned above. These may be online or offline groups. If you like to have some control in terms of decision-making, you may like groups like Weight Watchers or Edwards Diet. On the other hand, if you like to have meals prepared for you, you may consider groups like Nutrisystem from which you can order meals directly.

Do not Ignore Your Bones, Eyes, Ears or Screening Tests (BEES)

Do not ignore your bones, eyes, ears or screening tests? I say this because most people do not think about their bones, eyes, ears or screening tests (BEES), when they think about their health. Yet if we do not take care of our BEES, our health will eventually get stung.

I guess I should leave the jokes to the comedians. Did you know that osteoporosis is a disease characterized by low bone mass and fragile skeletons? This can lead to fractures of bones from falls or slips in the house as we get older.

Falling and having a hip fracture can quickly change a person's lifestyle from an independent freely moving adult, to one dependent on others to carry out the most basic activities of daily living like using the restroom.

This can lead to intense sadness, which may make an elderly patient unable to participate confidently in social activities. Without intervention loneliness and sadness could lead to depression.

Did you know that about 14% of people between 45 to 65, have some form of hearing loss? Why is this important for your health? This is important because not hearing well could make you become less engaging with people. You may find that each time you talk to people, you have to raise your voice or ask others to repeat themselves. This could lead to even the simplest things like going to the groceries becoming a very stressful activity.

Instead of trying to ignore people because of the associated stress, do not ignore your poor hearing or other ear symptoms. Go and see your doctor or health care provider and tell him or her about it.

As we get older our bodies begin to slow down and we sometimes become overwhelmed by all we have to do, just to keep up. If you have had good eye sight throughout your life, you may assume it will be there for life. However, soon you begin to realize that some eye diseases like cataracts, glaucoma, and macular degeneration occur as we get older.

Poor vision is not easy to deal with, it can lead to one's inability to read nutrition facts or even sign checks to pay for bills. This type of situation can be stressful, and we all know stress can be very bad for our health. Worst still, not seeing well can also lead to falls at home by tripping over furniture or other objects lying around the house.

Do not forget to go for your recommended screening tests. For women more than 50 years of age, most experts and specialists agree that getting a mammogram done can help detect breast cancer at their early and treatable stage. A mammogram is a special type of x-ray of the breast.

Everyone above 50 should be screened for colorectal cancer.If you are above 50 with an average risk of cancer, screening will entail doing stool testing annually, sigmoidoscopy or virtual colonoscopy every five years or colonoscopy every 10 years.

A screening test that has played a major role in reducing the number of women suffering from cervical cancer is the pap smear. It is a test most women are encouraged to start at age 21 or earlier if the are sexually active. This is a relatively simple test, but a few women refuse to do it for reasons best known to them.

A mother tearfully shared the story of her beautiful 35-year- old daughter, Jane, who died of cervical cancer in 2008 because she had decided not to have a pap test, so her cancer was diagnosed at a terminal stage. Her daughter said she could not bring her self to strip down for a test she felt she did not need. She considered the whole process too embarrassing and still refused the test even when she started having irregular menstrual bleeding.

Each time I think of Jane, tears well up in my eyes. I sincerely hope that anyone who reads her story will find out more about screening tests and do what test recommendations fit their circumstance.

Believe you me, your Bones, Eyes, Ears and Screening tests are an important part of healthy living and are strongly recommended in the Compass Health Transformer System. For more details on other recommended screening tests visit the U.S.Preventive Services Task Force website.

Do not ignore your finances

I know it is unusual to include finances when you are talking about healthy living, but the truth is that everything is interconnected. This is why I talk of the triangle of happiness founded on relationships, finances and health.

Remember that we need money to buy healthy food, to go to the laboratory for tests or doctor's visits, go to the movies and even to sign up for gym membership. Not having finances to pay your rent or your mortgage could result in losing your home. How easy will it be for you to take care of your health if you are homeless?

When you are examining your ambition and self knowledge profile, you should be honest with yourself on how much you earn and how you will spend it. This important source of stress cannot be overestimated. Some people have gone to bed and died during the night because of financial worries.

The state of your finances or unstable financial situation could significantly affect your ability to implement your individualized compass health plan. If you are concerned about your finances, talk to a financial expert or talk to trusted friends and family members who have a track record of handling their finances well. Do not talk to someone you do not trust because some scam artists will only make matters worse.

At least having a financial plan will help to reduce the stress that comes from not knowing what to do. The case of my patient who suffered from sleepless nights made me to appreciate the link between finances and good health. Her problems started when those who were supposed to help her get a loan modification ruined her credit and almost cost her, her home.

Her life changed from having sound sleep every night to sleepless nights. When I used my findings in her comprehensive health assessment protocol to check her triangle of happiness, I found out about her financial worries. I told her that the first step she needed to take was to spend what little money she had smartly and wisely. For example, I told her she could start saving money by buying things with coupons more regularly.

Of course, I also strongly encouraged her to see a financial expert to resolve her financial worries. I cannot give you details of what her own financial plan was, but I know that she resolved her financial stress and had more peaceful sleep. Don't ignore your finances and learn to live within your means while planning for the future.

This approach will help you to cut down on stress, sleep more soundly and wake up more prepared to make your day great. Have a healthy and happy life.

www.ingramcontent.com/pod-product-compliance
Lightning Source LLC
Chambersburg PA
CBHW072326290526
45794CB00002B/759